A TRAVEL NURSE'S GUIDE

Brian Fleig

A Travel Nurse's Guide

Copyright © 2019 Brian Fleig

All rights reserved.

ISBN: 9781092417389

A Travel Nurse's Guide

To Pip Fleig

My 38 year old wife of 20 years, best friend, adviser, business partner, and soul mate Passed away in 2002 of Cancer..

She was a mother of 2, great graphic artist, webmaster, nurse, companion and all around pain in the ass.

She was creative, ambitious, free thinker, singer, mother and the best conversationalist I have ever known.

She hardly ever did what I wanted her to but she almost always did the right thing. I can't remember doing anything without her having a hand in it.

She never asked for too much and always gave more than enough. She was half of everything I did and was.

A Travel Nurse's Guide

CHAPTER ONE
Introduction

This is the part where I tell you who I am so you know who you're listening to. If you want to skip this part, you are indeed free to do so.

I graduated from college as a nurse in May of 1993 and started full time on a medical floor at Highland Hospital in Rochester New York. In March 1994 I talked an agency into using me for a travel assignment even though their policy was to hire only after one full year out of school. My wife had graduated the year before as a nurse, and we wanted to move to Florida from New York. Our genius plan was why not let our career pay the expenses for the actual move. Sometimes genius plans work.

A Travel Nurse's Guide

Our first travel assignment went off as intended, and we ended up in New Port Richey Florida in March 1994. There was a fully furnished two bedroom apartment waiting for us complete with jobs. We drove there in our own vehicle and were paid mileage. I'm not even sure travel agencies were paying for flights in those days. In my five or so years in Florida, I ended up doing all kinds of different things, most of it either as per diem or through local staffing agencies. My wife herniated 2 disks (and I mean blew them out) on the job, so her career as a nurse was pretty much done although I didn't know it until a year or two later. My next travel assignment was moving the four of us back to New York, and I won't bore you with the long story, but we ended up in Syracuse.

Skipping ahead some more, I did my first strike in 1999, for the money. I was hooked. I spent the next year and 1/2 or so doing strikes full-time followed by the two of us starting our own travel nurse agency. The agency actually worked out very well even though we had no idea what we were doing, however a year into the agency was when my wife was diagnosed with cancer.

That was the beginning of the business's downhill slide. Moving ahead to December 2002, I was on my emotional feet, and although shaky I had to get back out making money, and the agency was closed. I didn't have the heart even to try reviving it after almost a year of chemo and radiation appointments. My first strike was in Hawaii in December 2002 and served as a launch pad for years straight travel assignments, with a smattering of per diem staff gigs in between. During all that time I had worked just about every area in the hospital, there was to work. I was never an ICU nurse, but I did a few shifts as a float, I was never an OB/GYN nurse either, but I did one shift as a float there too. I had done home healthcare, hospice, IV team and every kind of MedSurg you could name.

I've been full-time in the emergency room from 2003 to the present. During my time working emergency departments, I have worked four or five Trauma Centers in addition to numerous hospitals where the emergency department was no bigger than 4 beds and every size hospital in between. I have worked in eight or nine states and am licensed in even more. My last travel assignment was just over two years ago and am currently working as a house supervisor on staff in New York.

Travel nursing is a career in itself. In fact, it's a full-blown lifestyle. It's not just something that you make a phone call, and off you go, it takes a lot of work to get it off the ground. Once that work is done though, it's done. A lot of the set up is one time only and from there on every contract you take gets more comfortable because you get better at it. If you are sitting there thinking about how much you'd love this lifestyle, but you're coming up with reasons you can't do it, ask yourself a few questions.

Are my objections legitimate?

Are my objections based on fear of the unknown?

Do I want this lifestyle badly enough to make the effort?

P.S. Age is not an excuse. I have known a bunch of travelers in their 50s and 60s, myself being one of them.

If you want to do it, then do it. It is an adventure and adventure is admittedly not for everyone. Some people need safe and predictable, and that's okay. In this book, I will be leaning on a couple of current travel nurse friends for different perspectives, but the majority perspective is my own. Your mileage may vary.

CHAPTER TWO
Why Travel Nursing?

If you are not a travel nurse already, I believe the first thing you need to do is ask yourself what you want to get out of it is. There is any number of reasons you might want to be a travel nurse. For me, it was two reasons independence and money. I will talk more about independence in the next chapter. As a travel nurse, you can live where it's cheap and work where the pay is high. The whole country is literally your oyster. That's probably why so many travel nurses come from the deep South and end up going where the pay is high which is mostly California.

Maybe you just want to see the country. Well, this is an excellent way to do that and have it pay rather than cost. I would always get to my travel assignment early by a couple of days so that I could drive around, get the lay of the land and mostly make sure I had the route down pat from my hotel to the hospital. On the other end of the contract, I would stay an extra week and do my sightseeing. If you kept your work schedule down to three 12 hour shifts per week, you could sightsee the entire time you're there. I preferred to work five shifts a week sometimes six and then do my sightseeing at the end.

Another favorite reason for traveling for me was avoiding the corporate crap. As a traveler you do not have mandatory staff meetings, you're not being invited to join committees, there is no clinical ladder or whatever other buzzwords they have come up with for that. It bears mentioning, as a staff nurse it could take you years to get to the top of the pay scale via their ridiculous clinical ladders. As a travel nurse, you walk in the door at the top of the pay scale every time. And last but not least there is no he said she said backbiting bullshit. No one knows your business, you're not seeing your patients, and their family members in the grocery store and that girl/guy who dated your spouse in high school does not work in dietary. It's just plain awesome.

The way I did travel nursing was like I said earlier, I would go to a contract and work as many shifts as I could physically stand and that they would let me. When I worked strikes, I did seven days a week as most of us did. My record was 30 straight shifts. I've known other people who worked 40 to 90 consecutive shifts on strikes. You're probably not going be able to pull that off on a travel assignment. While working a strike you literally just eat sleep and work while they drive you back and forth. On a travel assignment, you're still going out to get your own meals, still taking the garbage out from your hotel room and dragging groceries into your room and driving yourself back and forth to work. All that stuff takes time and energy. However, it does not take nearly the amount of time and energy that all those things require at home. You don't have friends dropping over, you're not meal planning and grocery shopping for a week at a time because you're mostly eating out as a travel nurse. Anyway, I digress. The benefit I started off to tell you is that when you are off work, you are OFF work.

You're not off work three or four days a week, and you are not tired when you are off. You are off work for as long as you want to be off work. For as long as you can afford to be off work.

I traveled with my wife and kids at home, so I knew the house and the bills were being taken care of. When I was home in between assignments, I would take anywhere from 2 to 4 weeks off. I was there available for every event at the kids' school without losing sleep. I didn't have to come home from a 12-hour shift and then try to stay awake through a school play. I didn't have to miss a kids baseball game because of work. Obviously, I did miss those things when I was on contract, but I could also plan my contracts around the more important events. It's also possible, and I have done this, to schedule time off in the middle of a contract if you have an event that you don't want to miss. Obviously, if your contract is across the country from where you live, it's a transportation issue, but you should be able to afford it easily.

As much as I loved my travel nursing career, I will be honest and say it was not all unicorns rainbows and kittens. One of the downsides, at least for me, was loneliness. Although when I think about it, the isolation was after my wife was gone and my kids were grown up. Coming home to an empty house in between contracts was depressing. On the other hand, it was kinda neat. The house was exactly the way I left it which is actually pretty cool. I didn't have to come home after every contract either, I could go from contract to contract with a few weeks in between sightseeing. Back to loneliness, if you're a social butterfly and belong to bowling leagues or have friends over for barbecues every weekend, then loneliness could be an issue. You will miss out on a lot of that stuff. For me, that was not an issue, but if you think that might be an issue for you, then it is something you have to deal with. Lucky for me my personality has always leaned towards being a loner, in fact, most of the time I thrive on it. I need to circle back here though to how great it is when you are home to be home for two or three weeks at a time and have money to do anything you want.

    I have already touched on it here but let's cover one of the most significant objections I hear from people who want to be a travel nurse but are afraid to try it. I hear it all the time, "oh I wish I could be a travel nurse." My question to them is "why can't you be?" Their answer, 99 times out of 100, is that they have a spouse and have kids and can't leave them home alone. Again my question is "why can't you?" I did it for three or four years. Maybe it's easier for the male to leave the wife home with the kids versus the wife leaving the husband home with the kids. I can't answer that one. But I can say it is possible, I did it. Those years were not horrible, and when I was home, I was really home, unlike people that work three to five days every week. I can not even imagine ever going back to eight-hour shifts and a five day work week. I don't know how anybody does that and thinks they have any kind of home life.

    Personally, I think the biggest obstacle for people wanting to become a travel nurse is fear. Not everyone can venture into the unknown especially regularly. I'm actually glad that's the case because if everyone did it, then it wouldn't be as unique as it is. Which brings me to another downside of travel nursing although for me it's not a downside. Assuming most of your contracts are 13 weeks which is the standard these days, you will be in a brand-new environment three or four times per year. That means going through orientation, learning what might be new protocols although they don't really vary that much and learning to drive around a new city. One of the big ones probably is just learning a whole bunch of new names. Depending on whether you work at small hospitals or big trauma centers you could be learning 25 or 30 new names, and that's not a tiny thing. As a byproduct of this career for me, I find that I'm really terrible at remembering people's names. I think that's because I never made too much of an effort to memorize names. By the time I learn names I'm on my way out.

Some people will want to beat me up for this, but I still list this as a benefit. By the time management comes to you to nitpick about your charting or whatever else they want to nitpick over you're already gone. Although I have worked at one or two places where management was sharp enough to get their nitpicking in early. When I complain about nitpicking the first thing that comes to my mind was one place I worked in Nevada. They would come to me and complain I did not document the time that every patient was taken to and returned from radiology. That bothered me because it felt like they wanted me to document what the radiologist tech did. The tech came and did their own transports which was great but it's not like I was sitting there watching for them to come, I had my own job to do which did not include watching them. I didn't know what time they got there nor did I care. Why should I document what they do? One of my pet peeves I guess.

To summarize why you should ask yourself why travel nursing because it directs how you manage your career as a traveler. One of the things you'll have to do to get started obviously is getting licensed in other states which I will cover in another chapter. If you're in it primarily for the money, you probably want to focus on California because not only does that tend to be the highest paying state but they also have the highest volume of needs. If you're in it for the sightseeing, obviously you will want to get licensed in states that you want to see. If your goal is to see as much of the country as you can, then you need to plan out your licensing because some states require verifications from every state you've been licensed in. That may not be as big a problem these days because of online license verification that covers most states. Back in my day, I had to mail in a paper form with a $20 fee for every verification. More on that later.

    Another benefit of travel nursing is the pay scale. Too many hospitals nowadays are doing sliding pay scales based on years of experience. Personally, I think this is a scam. Once you hit that two-year mark, you are absolutely independent and are doing the same job that the person that's been there 10 or 12 years is doing. Why should you be making less money? At any rate, as a traveler, you are always at the top of the pay scale. Unlike years ago you may or may not be making more money than the staff nurses that you are working with, but you are at the top of the pay scale.

CHAPTER THREE

Best states to work in

I have worked in New York, Florida, New Hampshire, New Jersey, Ohio, Minnesota, Nevada, Arizona, California, and two islands in Hawaii. People sometimes ask me where was the best place to work. There is no simple answer to that. I will say that in my opinion, the best place to work in terms of pay rate is in California. Other than that I think it just boils down to what you want or expect from the experience. Vegas is incredible, obviously a fun place and it also pays pretty well. Hawaii is obviously awesome too, but it's so expensive to live there you'll probably be lucky to break even when you leave. That being said I do believe it's worth doing at least one assignment in Hawaii if you're a full-blown travel nurse. Who wants to be a 70-year-old old retired Nurse sitting in a rocking chair regretting not having gone to Hawaii for three months and breaking even doing it?

I have never been to Alaska, and I somewhat regret it. I have only known one nurse that took an assignment to Alaska, and he went for six months. His summary when he came back was he was glad he did it but would never do it again. I don't recall where he went in Alaska, but his most significant take away was dealing with the darkness. He was from Vegas, so I suppose it was extra hard coming from a sunny desert with an average annual rainfall of 5 inches and going to a snow-covered environment with extended darkness.

Back to working in California. My first assignment in California was in the year 2000. That was before the California State Nurses Association or whatever they call themselves forced through a ratio law. I was working on a MedSurg floor somewhere in San Bernardino when that law actually took effect. And yes the hospitals complied, and the ratios dropped, but the hospitals got their revenge.

Along with fewer patients we also had fewer ancillary staff. They took away CNAs, Housekeeping and cut back on Respiratory Therapy. That was what I most noticed at least. I'm pretty sure the end result of that was more work not less, but years later things are back to normal with the lower staffing ratios but then again by that time I was working in the ER which always was a ratio of 4 to 1. All in all, as much as I hate the political environment in California, I have to admit it is the easiest and the highest paying state to work in.

Las Vegas was mostly decent to work in, but I only worked ER there. I hated working in Reno, and there was one hospital that I would never work at again in Vegas. My favorite hospital to work at in Vegas was UMC.

I worked at two different hospitals in Arizona. One was quite nice, and the other was the nightmare from hell, both were in the ER. The nice one was in Tucson, and the nightmare from hell was called Valley or Desert View or whatever in Fort Mohave which is up near the corner of Nevada and California. The same company that owned the Valley Hospital also owned the hospital in Lake Havasu Arizona and based on what I heard from many different people that also was the nightmare from hell to work at.

Another point worth mentioning is that most hospitals on the West Coast, at least that I was exposed to, are for-profit hospitals. That is also true for Florida, while the hospitals I've worked at in the Northeast were all not-for-profit. You would think that Non-profit would equal better, but that is not always the case. There is one hospital in New York that I would put in the top five worst places I have ever worked. The one I'm talking about in New York was a 16 bed ER with four nurses plus a triage nurse plus a charge nurse. The charge nurse did not take patients. The triage nurse came back and helped when there were no triages which wasn't usually till well after midnight. The charge nurse tried to help when he or she could but was generally busy without doing any patient care. That staffing was decent, but the problem came when someone called in sick.

Any other ER I have worked in would close four beds when someone called in sick. But in this place, they just gave you more patients. It was not uncommon to have five or six and one or two of those could potentially be a very sick ICU type patient that took up most of your time. Very dangerous practice in my opinion. Based on what I heard from other travelers that was a standard thing around smaller hospitals in Central New York. I should mention that I am not talking about New York City, I have never worked in a hospital in New York City and never will.

In Hawaii, I worked on two different strikes. One of them was at Queen's Medical Center on Oahu, in December 2002, which is a level I trauma center. At that facility, I worked on a Neuro ICU step down floor. Remember, it's best to be flexible so that you are perceived as valuable. That one was a pretty awesome experience. Sometime in 2004 or maybe it was 2005, I did a strike on the island of Kauai. That one sucked, but I won't bother to go into details why. I made great money at Queens but only because I worked 30 straight 12 hour shifts. The overtime has always been where you make the money on strikes.

Had I been paying my own hotel bill and only working three shifts a week I would have been lucky to get out of there breaking even. When I was done with the strike at

Queens a female ICU nurse, and I went to Maui and spent a week in a condo. All in all one of the best experiences of my life.

CHAPTER FOUR
Do's and Don'ts

I strongly recommend you have two years of nursing experience before you attempt travel nursing. Most agencies have a rule of one year, but my experience has been that two years makes you a much stronger nurse which means much less stress dropping yourself into a brand-new environment.

DO take care of yourself. You have probably heard the mantra "take good care of your tools." In this case, you are the tool, and I don't mean that in a derogatory, insulting way. If you need new shoes get 2 pairs in case, one ends up pinching you. Don't skimp on comfortable clothes and that includes socks and underwear. If you need a Velcro knee brace go to a pharmacy and buy one. If you need new glasses buy two or three pairs, so you have backups. Your body is the most critical tool in your toolbox to maximize your career, take care of it.

DO carry your complete file with you at all times. I cannot stress this enough. The agency and/or the hospital WILL lose items out of your file and request another copy from you. Of course, they will play it like you never sent it to them in the first place. Equally important: Make sure you get and keep (and carry with you) a copy of everything, including all up to date medical stuff. TB test, Physical, Chest X-ray, Flu shot, etc. If the agency pays for you to go get a Flu shot or Physical or whatever make sure you get a copy from the place that does it. If they refuse to give you a copy because you didn't pay for it, then plan on getting your own done at some point. When you check in to a hotel 1,000 miles from, and the agency says they lost a part of your medical record good luck getting a new physical on Friday for a Monday start date. The one exception to that is pre-employment drug screens. You'll never get a copy of that and even if you do no one will accept your copy anyway.

DO bring 7 days of scrubs, if you can, and 2-3 sets of non-scrubs. The less often you have to do laundry the better.

DO invest in a GPS if you don't already have one in your car or on your phone.

DO consider a laptop if you depend on your computer. Setting up a desktop in a hotel room is mostly a non-starter.

DO consider a large data plan on your smartphone. WiFi in most hotels is terrible. Setting your phone up as a hotspot works great if you have the data to cover it. I have streamed hour-long TV shows using my Verizon phone and a laptop, and it was as smooth as watching it on TV.

DO Get your own health insurance. I could buy a policy in Nevada as an individual all day, at least pre Obamacare. In NY not so much, but with a $25 business license from the county clerk I was able to get a policy through the local Chamber of

Commerce.

DO be willing to float to other areas of the hospital. Floating will probably be a rare event as a traveler, but the more flexible you are, the more valuable you are. If you have absolutely no experience working in ICU and they send you to the ICU go to the ICU. Walk into the ICU and say: "I am not an ICU nurse, but I will do what I can to help." You will be a hero in addition to being exposed to new experiences that you may never have otherwise had.

DO get certs even if you don't need them. Mainly, I am talking about ACLS and PALS even if you work someplace where you don't need those, any certifications you have move you towards the top of the hiring list. That's true for staff as well as travelers. If you work in the ER try to get TNCC (Trauma Nurse Core Course) and ABLS (Advanced Burn Life Support). And of course, there is always CEN for ER, CCRN for ICU, Certified Diabetic Educator and many more. I know CEN and CCRN are rather ridiculous to get in terms of cost and time spent studying but the more certifications you have, the more perceived value you have.

DO NOT forget the little things. Cell phone charger, laptop, Kindle device, toiletries, your favorite coffee mug, etc. It goes without saying I know but write yourself a list and follow it. I can't tell you how many cell phone chargers I've bought at truck stops over the years. I bring my own alarm clock because some hotel alarm clocks aren't all that easy to figure out or just plain don't work.

DO NOT tell the staff of the hospital where you are going how you did things at home. You are not there to change anything, you are there to blend in and help out. They don't care how you did it where you came from. Chances are pretty good that there will be times when it's appropriate to share your past experiences but be very sparing with it.

DO NOT be the person who thinks the way you originally learned it is the only way it can or should be done. Flexibility in this career is a big key to success as well as your own mental health.

DO NOT expect a full-blown orientation like you would have with a staff position. Even hospitals that go overboard, or what I consider as overboard, on orientation limit it to five days in the classroom and then possibly two or three days with a preceptor. I talk my way out of that crap. It's understandable to spend a day or two in a computer lab if it's software that you've never used before but beyond that one shift with a preceptor is what I try to talk my way in to. And don't be afraid to try convincing them to schedule your precept shift(s) at night if you work nights. Why do they all assume that everyone MUST precept on day shift? Also, how do people wake up that early every morning?

DO NOT Take anything personally. Nod your head smile and walk away. If you don't already have a thick skin, grow one. There are still bitter staff nurses out there who resent us for making what they think is a million dollars a week.

CHAPTER FIVE
Independence

Hopefully one of your motivating factors for jumping into this career is to feel as independent as you can. Travel nursing is the ideal vehicle for feeling independent short of running your own business. Then again, as a business owner how much vacation time they get to take.
Independence though is something you will have to take, no one is going to hand it to you.

The reason I say that is that agencies vary dramatically in how they treat you and how they pay you. Years ago I called them the evil Empire which included Travcor, American mobile, Cross Country and a few others. Those companies were ridiculously low pay and treated you like you were an idiot. I have to admit though to being an idiot as a newbie traveler. Maybe idiot is the wrong word, I mean they held your hand in every junction like they did not want you even to know it was possible to be independent. They had a nice furnished apartment for you to stay in and they would call you every two days to ask you how it was going. I suppose that was to make sure your feelings weren't hurt, or you weren't freaking out being in a new city or whatever. On the other end of that spectrum are the companies that pay the best but are not paying a ridiculous amount of office staff to hold your hand. They will not put you in a fancy apartment with a centerpiece of flowers waiting for you on the dining room table. They will put you in a hotel room, usually an extended stay hotel room but not always. They will not call you regularly and drive you crazy because they expect you to be a grown-up adult who can manage your own life.

    Some people would say that I took independence to the extreme. I knew a few people that went even farther than I took it. I will tell you how I managed my career in terms of independence, and you can decide how far you want to go. Let me start by explaining how a typical travel contract with a typical agency goes. I'm not talking one of the hand holding crappy pay agencies either. Typically you will sign up with an agency, spend hours filling out forms and send in all your stuff to build your file. You probably already know this, but your file includes your application your skills checklist year a copy of your TB test of physical, etc. Etc. By the way, fax machines are mostly dead technology, nowadays you need a scanner and email to submit all this stuff.

Once your file is built, then you will talk to your recruiter who you hopefully get along well with, and discuss the availability of contracts where you want to go. So your recruiter says I have a hospital in XYZ California that is paying $55 an hour for three 12 hour shifts per week are you interested? By the way, all travel shifts that I am aware of are 12 hours. It is not worth your time to do eight-hour shifts in this career. So you say yes please submit me to that hospital. The recruiter takes your file and transmits it to whomever it may concern at that hospital. Then usually the department manager of wherever it is that you've been submitted to whether it's MedSurg or ER or whatever will call you on the phone for a phone interview. In the phone interview, the manager will explain to you what the unit is like and how many shifts they expect from you. They will probably ask you questions about your skills and your background. Just relax and be yourself.

They will not tell you anything negative in a phone interview, it's up to you to read between the lines on that score. I end every phone interview with the question, "what is your nurse to patient ratio?" In California, it's never an issue; however some places it is. The national standard whether it's written or unwritten for an ER nurse is four patients to one nurse. When the answer to that question starts with "we try" or "usually" that's a huge red flag to me.

My point here is that you really have to read between the lines and you get better at it with experience. And don't be afraid to ask them whatever question pops into your head. Also, the phone interview is the absolute best time to bring up any scheduling issues you might have. For example, if one of your kids has a championship baseball game or your sister is getting married in the middle of your future contract, and you want to fly home to see it. The phone interview is the best time to bring that up, then follow up on it when you get there. It's best to bring it up in the phone interview so that there's no question before you even leave your house. It's important to remember that they will not mistreat you in most cases, but they will not treat you the same as their staff nurses either. Without being confrontational, you have to be assertive in getting what you need.

So all that has gone well, and you've accepted the assignment. You've set a start date with the agency and/or in the phone interview. To get there, either they're going to pay you mileage to drive, or they're going to fly you. Most of the time nowadays they want to fly you, especially if it's cross-country but the rental car once you are there is going to be on you. Or they might put you in housing that will be convenient, you hope, to public transportation assuming the hospital is a city. Personally, I can't stand public transit, then again who wants to deal with driving in downtown DC, Denver, NYC, etc.?

Rental cars are overpriced and an expense I hate to pay for.

If you do do the rental car thing, you usually get a better rate if you do 30 days at a time by the way. So you fly into the city and get a cab or shuttle or whatever to your hotel. Hopefully, you are there a day or two early so that you can learn your way around and stock your hotel room with whatever snacks and drinks you want. That is zero independence on a scale of 0 to 10 based on my perspective.

Here's how I would prefer to handle it. Before the agency ever submits me for a contract they know I will manage my own transportation, housing, health insurance, etc. I do NOT want their benefits. I don't want them doing anything for me other than connecting me to a contract. Nothing makes you less independent than being tied to an employer by the "benefit" tendril.

Before I even have a phone interview I've already gone online and found hotels in the area of the contract so that I could research pricing, how nice they are, and what kind of neighborhoods they are in. More than once I have ended up telling the agency either cancel my submission or don't submit me because there just are no viable hotel options for that particular hospital. The reason I do this is that I want the maximum dollars per hour in my paycheck. Everything the agency does for you will come out of your paycheck; you just won't see it. It comes out in the form of fewer dollars per hour.

One benefit of doing it this way is that you can write off the hotel bills, rental car bills, food, etc. on your taxes assuming you itemize. For me, the benefit is I just want to be in control of my own housing, I might not want to stay in the super eight that they put me in. I might want to stay in a Hilton this time and then the next contract I might want to stay in a super eight. The other thing I do is drive to the contract. The first few years I did the flying thing and public transportation. Then I graduated to a rental car, but I got really sick of the whole flying trauma. I don't mind the flying itself, but the airport hassle just got to be stupid post 911.

Another reason to drive yourself is something you don't think about until you're facing the hard truth. When you're on an assignment whether you do your sightseeing during your work schedule or afterward you're going to buy stuff and good luck getting it home on an airplane. I've bought wall hangings, clothes, shoes and all kinds of stuff that I could not fit in my luggage, and so has everyone else I've known.

You will get paid mileage to drive, and I don't think I've ever lost money in terms of what I spent on gas. If you include wear and tear on your car then maybe you lose money driving, but that's the price I was willing to pay for independence. Another option that I've done a couple of times is to rent a car at home and drive it to the assignment. Not the best financial option but it saves you wear and tear on your own vehicle.

Another benefit to booking your own hotel room aside from getting the neighborhood and the price range that you want is you get to make sure you get a room with a refrigerator or microwave or whatever features you want in that room. I would much rather be the one responsible rather than leaving it to someone who may or may not care. I say that's a benefit because too many times whoever made the booking at the travel agency either didn't care or was too busy, or whatever but I got none of the features that I wanted. When you live in a room for three months, those features are important. If you work the night shift, don't forget to tell them that you want a room as far away from the ice machine the elevator and a stairway door as you can get.

CHAPTER SIX
Licensing

There is really not a whole lot to be said about licensing. No matter what state you are licensed in you can get a license in every other state, it's just a matter of filling out paperwork and of course paying the fee. Go to Google and search for the state nursing board for where you want to go then find their licensing page. Every state's website, of course, is a little different but it's not that hard to navigate around. The only tricky part is the few states who want verification from every state you have ever been licensed in. To my knowledge, those states are Massachusetts, New Jersey, Michigan and I'm thinking maybe Illinois. I could be wrong on those but be aware.

My suggestion would be to sit and consider what states you think you might ever want to travel to and go research what it takes to get a license in each of those states. The reason is, if you think you might want to travel to Massachusetts and that state requires verifications of from every state you've ever been licensed in you'll want to do that first while you only have one or two licenses. It just simplifies the process. Now in this day and age, you have https://www.nursys.com/ for verifications, but I don't think every state participates. I could be wrong about this you'll have to look into it. I have used nursys to look up my own licenses for entertainment purposes, but I had never used it for verifications because it was not yet widely used when I obtained all my licenses.

The other thing you need to be aware of is the nursing license compact. My understanding has always been that the NCLEX is the NCLEX regardless of what state you take it in. If the test is the same in every state why in the hell do we have to apply for a separate license in every state? Well, the answer is money. So the nursing compact is an agreement between states to recognize the license from the other states in the compact and it has been growing for years. To see where it stands go here https://www.ncsbn.org/nurse-licensure-compact.htm

Technically, you have to live in one of the compact states to be eligible to work in the other compact states. For example, I currently live in New York, but I have an Arizona license. When I lived in Arizona, I could work in any of the compact states without getting a license in that state. Now that I live in New York even though I still have an Arizona license I cannot work in a compact state without getting a license in that state. I know, it is stupid. I know of a couple people who have snuck around that by getting a drivers license in a compact state when they didn't live in that state. The DL and a mailing address are all the Board of Nursing wants to see for proof of residence. Of course, you have to get a PO Box or some other type of residence in that state to get mail and a drivers license. I assume they probably frown on that practice, I don't know, but if you're desperate, I have heard that it works. Hey, it's not like you lose your nursing skills based on what state you live in.

A final word on licensing, some states

are simple and other states are a real pain in the ass. Just to be on the safe side plan on 3 to 6 months to get a license. Some states have temporary licenses for an extra fee, and some states don't. Some states are what they call, and some states are not. Walk-through means that you can walk into the Board of Nursing office with all your paperwork (already filled out) and they will process you right then and there, for a temporary license. Personally, I think depending on a walk-through is a dangerous practice. If you drive across three states on Wednesday to start a job on Monday and you're depending on that walk-through to work things could go wrong fast. Think about it. You will be at the mercy of bureaucrats who really don't care if you get your license or not. They may be working at half staff because of sick calls. They may be closed for some stupid state holiday that you didn't even know existed. They may just have a bad attitude that day. Think of the worst day you ever had at a DMV and remember this could just as easily happen in a state licensing office. On the other hand, it could go flawlessly, I just don't recommend you banking on it. The bottom line is if you plan on going to a particular state to work you better start working on a license long before you think about going there.

CHAPTER SEVEN
Finding Agencies

Most recruiters are really good at their job. But the truth is that it's not a skilled position, it's a learn on the job position. I suppose there really is no other job quite like it that you could call previous experience. Having employed recruiters when I owned my own agency I believe that it's hard for them making what they make while serving people that make three or four times more. Basically, they are your personal secretary in as far as it takes for you to get a job.

Another thing I learned owning my own agency is that there are a lot of whiny ass travel nurses out there who think they deserve the world and lay it all on their recruiter in the form of bad attitude. Don't be that person. There is nothing wrong with trying to get the world but give your recruiter a break.

I will list a few agencies in a collection of resources at the end of this book. Google is your friend in this regard. You may find a decent agency in the back of one of the nursing magazines, but I'd be willing to bet not. I personally would stay away from the agencies in the magazines. Then again I haven't read a nursing magazine in years so I could be wrong. I think every agency I've ever signed up with, and there has been at least a dozen for me, I have learned about from other travelers. In all the years I did travel I was never active with less than three agencies at any given time because it's really great getting regular text messages and emails with different pay rates and locations.

That brings me to another topic. I have been vocal about this over the years with the agencies that I've worked for, not that it always helps. I would tell them not to bother sending me job postings without pay rates. And what really pisses me off is the agencies that won't tell you the pay rate when you call them. It's happened to me more than once where I will call them based on an email they sent me, and they will want me to catch up on expired items in my file before they talk pay rates. Or perhaps this was an agency I never worked for, and they got my email address somewhere, and they would not tell me pay rates until after I filled out a complete file. Not going to happen. My standard answer to that was why would I spend my time filling out your paperwork if you can even be bothered to tell me a pay rate? Then in other cases, they won't immediately tell you the pay rate because they have to apply some convoluted mathematical algorithm. Another big red flag for me.

When they try to pull this smoke and mirrors tax deferment this and that bullshit, I will tell them, just give me your best hourly rate. I will take care of transportation housing and everything else, just give me your best hourly rate. If they still try to work with the smoke and mirrors bullshit, I'm moving on. No time for nonsense. My thought is that the hospital, the patient's, and even the agencies expect me to be forthcoming honest and true to my word. I damn sure expect the same in return. If you can't just name a pay rate, it makes me think you're trying to run some kind of scam. Maybe I'm being overly sensitive, but I don't care, there are too many options out there to put up with nonsense. Okay, I am done with my soapbox.

So ideally you will start off with two or three agencies which will probably take an entire weekend at home filling out paperwork because the file requirements over the years have just gone off the chart. It's worth it though. It's also an excellent idea to always keep your ears open for recommendations of any new agencies. There's a lot of agencies out there that only deal with certain types of contracts or certain hospitals or whatever. I have fallen into a couple niches just by keeping my ears open.

One example is Coalinga California. There was only one agency serving this hospital, and I can't even remember where I found out about it. It was one of the best travel deals I ever got. I lived in Vegas at the time, so I was about a 6-hour drive from the hospital. It was so small that it only took one RN per night shift in the ER. What they did was schedule three RNs per month to cover night shift working 10 consecutive night shifts each. The agency rented a three-bedroom house three or 4 miles away from the hospital. It was perfect because each of us had our own bedroom and we could leave clothes or bedding or whatever we wanted to in the bedroom and always come back to the same bedroom. I would arrive at the house one day before my first of 10 shifts and the next day the nurse that I was replacing would leave to drive home. I would not have anyone else in the house until the last day of my shift when my replacement showed up. They paid $6500 for 10 shifts which obviously is $650 per shift, and then they charged us $500 each for the rent on the house which included furniture, cable TV, Wi-Fi for Internet, pots, and pans, etc. It was a fully functional turnkey house for us. We were not required to use their house but $500 per month for a full house with a full kitchen was a lot better than any hotel room, so that was a no-brainer. When I got home after my 10 shifts, I had 20 days off and could have easily worked a per diem job at home and made another few thousand dollars. Sadly though I did not do that.

The point is I would never have gotten that gravy job if I had not been listening and taking notes when other travelers talked. I would include the name of this particular agency at the end of the book, but I cannot remember it, it's been too many years.

CHAPTER EIGHT
Contracts

Length of available contracts is something that seems to cycle, probably based on desperation. When I first started traveling it was pretty standard to be able to get four-week contracts. You could get 13-week contracts back then, but it was just as easy to find a four week, six week, or eight week. I've always had the attitude as a traveler that you can do anything for 13 weeks. It's only three months, and it just gets exponentially easier for four weeks or six weeks or eight weeks. However, these days it's tough to find anything less than 13 weeks. They are still out there, but they're few and far between. I suspect once you have a relationship with an agency and ask them outright you might find that they have them. Agencies don't want to tell you because they put a lot of effort into getting you into a contract, so they want that contract to go on as long as possible to justify their effort.

Be an easy nurse to work with from the perspective of the agency and the hospital. Once the agency has placed you in two or more contracts if you're the one that's not whining, not complaining and you don't have 100 silly requests they will be more willing to open up contracts they might not otherwise even tell you about. Trust me on this, they don't want to give their best contracts out to nurses that are just a thorn in their side. Another possible thing, and I know because I've done it, is to ask the agency to submit you to a specific hospital on the condition that you can only work X number of weeks. You might be surprised how often that strategy works, but it starts with you being a joy for the agency to work with.

By being easy to place I mean you don't expect them to find housing for you that accepts Pets. Don't take your spouse and kids with you and expect them to find three or four bedroom housing. Don't have a bunch of oddball requests, either take the standard off-the-shelf deal or get independent and manage the housing and transportation on your own. Once an agency knows that you are easy to deal with, you're not a complainer, you don't quit on contracts, you don't miss your flight and need it rescheduled, you show up on time, and the hospital likes you then opportunities will start opening up.

On the flip side of that, I don't ever recommend signing up for a contract that's longer than necessary. In other words, if they are asking for eight weeks don't volunteer to sign up for 13 weeks. You can always extend, believe me, no one will ever say no to an extension. I say that because you never know, it could be a hellhole. There are only a few reasons hospitals use travelers in the first place. One of those reasons is it could be a hellhole that can't retain nurses. It has only happened a few times to me, but they are out there and sometimes "hellhole" is in the eye of the beholder.

I think out of, and I am guessing here, 60 or so contracts I've taken over the years I have only quit on two, that were so bad it just wasn't worth it for me to stay. And for me to abandon a contract, it was awful. Sometimes it's not so much that the hospital is terrible, but it's just a terrible fit for you.

That same logic applies to signing up for three shifts per week when that's offered. Don't volunteer for more shifts than they require before you get there and feel out the job. The likelihood is that you will be able to pick up as many shifts as you want to assuming the job goes well for you. It's twice as bad when you committed to four or five shifts per week upfront then you get there and find out you hate the job.

CHAPTER NINE

Transportation and Housing

A quick Google search shows that the IRS mileage reimbursement rate for business use in 2019 is $0.58 per mile up 3.5 cents from 2018. Every agency I have ever worked with uses the IRS rate for mileage reimbursement although they may have a per trip cap. This is very much worthwhile when you consider taking your own car to an assignment as opposed to flying. I drive a Ford half-ton pickup and average 18 miles per gallon which comes out to a reimbursement rate of $10 per gallon of gas. Even if you have to drive through the mountains and your fuel mileage is half that you're still way ahead of the game. Add to that your sense of freedom to come and go whenever you want, sightsee whenever you want and never have to pay for a rental car or cab and I believe driving your own vehicle to the assignment is a no-brainer. Now, of course, that assumes that you have a late model reliable car with good tires good brakes, etc. Don't drive a car a thousand miles if you are not sure that it will make it there.

I always try to have at least $3000 sitting in the bank to go start an assignment. That's the minimum amount I want to cover myself for transportation costs, upfront hotel costs and just in case costs. The two times I actually did quit assignments in the middle, or near the beginning really, I would not have made it home or to the next job if I had not had that buffer of cash. If you don't have a cushion of money then, by all means, start your travel career off taking their travel, housing and using public transportation or whatever you have to do. Work extra shifts to build that buffer. It is such a massive load off your mind knowing you have that buffer of cash (or available credit) and that nothing can hurt you. When I ran my agency, it amazed me how many travel nurses were perpetually broke and always asking for advances. It's not rocket science.

Bear in mind that if you choose the rental car option, you will most definitely want to rent that car for one week at a time and if the cost is $250 or $300 per week they're going to charge you the week in advance in addition to an equal amount for deposit possibly. The same goes for the hotel, in fact, the hotel may want to charge you for 30 days at a time, or it may just be that you get a much better rate if you pay for 30 days at a time. In either case, you better have cash or credit to cover that. Obviously, any time you drive long distance away from home you need to have some money or credit in case of breakdown also.

One last point on transportation that also comes back to independence. If you take company transportation such as a flight they may very well have booked you a return date before you even leave home. To save money, most flights that are booked by travel agencies are non-changeable. That means if you leave the assignment early for whatever reason family emergency, personal illness, can't stand the job, you may have to fight tooth and nail to get that agency to cover your flight home. They may refuse to cover your flight home I have heard of that happening. Also, if you fly on the company's dime not only will that be a couple dollars less that you're going to get per hour, but you have to cover cab fare to and from the airport on your own. You may or may not get reimbursed but either way, you have to cover it out of pocket upfront.

    I know I keep coming back to independence and freedom, but in my mind, that is the most significant selling point of a travel nurse career.

    Now for hotels. I always managed my own hotels after the first few assignments that I did. Long before you leave and possibly even before you accept the assignment, you should be finding yourself a hotel online. If it's a fair sized city that you're going to you don't have to worry about availability prior to accepting the contract, but if it's a small hospital in the middle of nowhere it could be an issue, and you better find out before you dive in. Anyway, I always preferred extended-stay hotels, but they are not always available. If you have to use a regular everyday hotel or motel call them up and find out about the availability of refrigerator and microwave.

If they do not have a microwave available and that is important to you, you can bring one with you from Walmart for 30 or 40 bucks if you're driving, or buy one when you get there. It's not quite as easy to carry a mini fridge with you though. Most hotels and motels only have a certain number of refrigerators which means fewer refrigerators than rooms. Some places have a fridge in every room, but that is the minority. If you have arranged ahead of time by phone to have a fridge in your room, but when you get there they tell you there are none available, which can happen, here is a trick. I have never used this trick myself, and honestly, I don't really like it, but I've seen other people use it. Tell them that you are diabetic and you need the refrigerator to keep your insulin. I know, and you know that insulin does not need to be refrigerated, but most people don't know that and they will magically come with a fridge. Meaning they will confiscate one from someone else. It's a dirty trick, but I've seen it work.

CHAPTER TEN
Portable Housing

Something a lot of travel nurses, including myself, dream of is to bring your own housing with you to every assignment. Wouldn't it be awesome to have your own bed, bedding, coffee maker, etc. with you away from home?

I considered it for many years and finally pulled the trigger on that in 2011. I bought a 31-foot motor home for $9000 that was about 20 years old. My logic was that I was going to see if I liked living in a motor home and what features I wanted or didn't like and then after a year or two I would upgrade to a new one. I took it as far as to move out of my rented house which was in

Arizona at the time and live in the motor home full time. Yes, I downsized everything, sold all my furniture and a lot more. It was actually quite painful, but I looked at it as a new adventure. Part of my thought process was that through the years I noticed that every place I had been had positives and negatives. I could not decide where I wanted to live, where I wanted my home base to be. The conclusion I came to was that if I lived in a motor home, I could purchase 1/4 acre or 1/2 acre lot in multiple states and set them all up with water, sewer and electric. Whatever state I was in the mood to live in I could pull on to my own lot and be home.

The experiment did not work out for me but for reasons that had nothing to do with the concept. A very good friend of mine has been following that concept for many years although she still maintains a home base. In Rachel's case, she and her husband travel by fifth wheel camper that they pull with a 1-ton diesel truck. Her husband is retired, so he maintains the camper and does most of the towing and stuff like that. I recently asked her if she would still do the trailer thing if it were just her. Her answer was absolutely yes with no hesitation. When I came up with my motor home plan, I thought it sounded like a real pain in the ass to have to disconnect a trailer so that you could use the truck to drive to the hospital from the campground. I suppose though it's no more of a pain than it would be to disconnect the car that you're pulling behind the motor home.

    I asked Rachel how her costs broke down for pulling the trailer versus using extended-stay hotels. She had done the math, and she included the payment for the truck because you definitely want a late model truck she included the payment for the trailer which is also late-model with the cost of the campground. She says it is definitely cheaper than a hotel room, some times significantly cheaper. And again the benefit of freedom and independence is enormous. The only downside that she could think of was that sometimes, especially in a city, you end up parking the camper 30 to 40 minutes away from the hospital. She does not mind the drive, and I certainly would not mind the 30 to 40-minute drive either. If that would be an issue for you, then that may not be the way to go. I imagine RV campgrounds are all on the outskirts of cities making for a 30+

minute drive to work for a contract in any medium to large city.

I believe she has her own washer and dryer in the camper which is probably small, but I would rather do numerous loads than pay three dollars per load on coin-op machines in the hotel that may or may not even work. The other benefit to bringing your own housing with you is the kitchen would save money over take out. That depends of course on being in a mood to cook if you're working four or five straight 12 hour shifts. If you want to maximize your income by working four or five or six shifts per week, develop yourself an overall routine that simplifies your life as much as possible. This may include eating at the hospital cafeteria or getting drive through on the way to work. Whatever it takes to create a lifestyle that's as stress-free as you can make it.

CHAPTER ELEVEN
Pay-Taxes-Banking

PAY

As I said earlier in this book some agencies will try to throw what I consider to be smoke and mirrors at you in the form of nontaxable stipends or whatever term they want to come up with for it. What it boils down to is they give you a base rate of something really low like 18 or 20 bucks an hour and then the balance of your pay is provided to you with different labels that they claim are nontaxable. Having owned an agency in the past, I can tell you that it is possible for the IRS to come after you for that money at some point because in their eyes it is still income and is still taxable.

With that being said, the IRS rules change every year so take that with a grain of salt. What you really want to beware of in a situation like that is if they set your pay scale up so that your base rate is 20 bucks an hour you better make sure your contract gives a full rate for overtime pay. You don't want time and 1/2 for overtime to be based on 20 bucks an hour. They haven't actually tried to pull that on me in quite a few years, but it has been pulled on me. The last few contracts that I have accepted under those conditions have included a paragraph that states the overtime rate is 60 bucks an hour or 55 an hour or whatever.

In California, you should probably not make less than 50 or $55 an hour and in some cases as much as $70 an hour. If you are on staff in California making $50 an hour, you will get time and 1/2 on $50 an hour which means every hour you work over 40 you make $75 so look over your contract carefully before you sign it.

Another term to beware of is "blended rate." I'm not sure anyone still does this, but it was big at one time. It is straight time, and over time blended together. For example, your contract is for 48 hours per week (4 shifts). They take the time and 1/2 for the 8 hours and "blend" it into your straight time. Even IF the math works out accurately, you lose on that deal if you work over 48 hours.

If you drive, you will get reimbursed for mileage, but you have to have gas money up front. If you get your own housing, you will get a monthly, what the agency calls housing stipend, although they will probably pay it weekly. By the way, all travel pay is weekly which is another big advantage of traveling versus working staff.

TAXES

I have heard from travelers for years that your tax guy has to know how to do taxes specifically for travel nurses. I personally don't believe that I think all you need is someone who knows how to file in different states because you do have to file in every state that you've worked. Here's another thing to be aware of if you do accept a contract where they break your pay into taxable and nontaxable. Bear in mind that the taxable amount will be the only thing that shows up on your W-2. While it's great not paying taxes on the full amount if you want to apply for a mortgage next year your W-2 is going to show half of what you actually made. And guess what the bank uses to qualify your mortgage. In other words, if they get your "taxable pay" down to $20/hour, you will qualify for a mortgage based on that $20/hour regardless of the fact your actual income may have been $50/hour.

Ask a tax guy what the ramifications might be if you do accept a contract with so-called nontaxable stipends. By the way, the agency is motivated to give you this nontaxable stipend because it gives them a significant break on their payroll tax expenses. However, if you get audited and the IRS decides you need to pay taxes on all or part of that tax-free stipend that's on you not on the agency so be careful.

BANKING

It's probably not necessary, but there may come a day when it's helpful for you to have a national bank. If you live on the East Coast and you work on the West Coast and absolutely have to get into your bank to fix some problem wouldn't it be nice to have a branch of your bank right down the street from your hotel? I had Bank of America for most of my travel days, and yes there were a few times that I absolutely had to get into a branch. Also, before you start driving your car cross-country filling the gas tank with your debit card call your bank and tell them that you will be driving cross country and filling your gas tank. If you don't, you will be sitting somewhere with an empty gas tank and a credit or debit card that has been shut off because they thought it was stolen. If that does happen, call the number on the back of the card. In the meantime, carry a few hundred $ in cash just in case.

Most people use direct deposit these days, but if you don't, it is a must for travelers. Unless your spouse is at home depositing your checks, you MUST have direct deposit. Yes, most agencies offer the option of sending your paycheck to your hotel via FedEx. Just a bad idea, do direct deposit. This is another good time to talk about having a cash buffer in the bank or in your pocket. If you get to your assignment on a shoestring, remember you won't be getting a check for two weeks. You have to work a week, and then you get paid the end of the following week, and that's if nothing goes wrong with either the check or the direct deposit. If there is a holiday in the pay processing week or someone drops the ball, and you are on a shoestring you're gonna go hungry.

CHAPTER TWELVE
Resources

My email address:
Brian@TheNursinginsider.com

Feel free to email me with comments, complaints, marriage proposals, questions, or invitations to barbecues.

Travel Nursing Forums / Blogs

https://www.thegypsynurse.com/blog/new-rn-ready-travelnurse/

https://forums.delphiforums.com/traveln

urses?gid=2138251909   I'm not a fan of this one but a lot of people are.

Http://www.MobileRN.com   This site is down as I write this, apparently for revamping. When it's up, it is frequented by long term travel and strike nurses. It hasn't been super active the last few years but worth a look now and then. It started as Scab.org which I started, but I sold it to Jon (can't recall his last name), and he dropped the scab label because he felt it had negative connotations. In its early years, it was getting as much as a half million hits per month and was covered by the LA Times, a nursing magazine and even CNN. I still remember how weird it was waking up in a hotel room on a strike years ago waiting for the coffee to brew and seeing my own website on CNN.

A pretty good article about travel nursing pay from Jan 2018

Agencies
Sunbelt staffing

Rapid Temps
Fastaff (Has a division that does strikes)
Health Source Global... They do travel and strikes.

MISC

https://www.aviatorscrubs.com/donsshop / Best scrubs money can buy but they are not cheap. They are made with the same or similar material as the flight suits that helicopter crews wear.

The following came to my email as I was putting the finishing touches on this book. May your text messages and emails be full of offers like this:

ER: Registered Nurse is needed in Mount Holly, NJ !

SKILLS NEEDED: having experience with EPIC is a plus

SHIFT: (10:00am – 10:30pm) or (7:00am

– 7:30pm)

REQUIREMENTS: Current NJ RN License, previous ER experience

CERTIFICATIONS: ACLS, BLS, PALS

START: April 23rd 2019

PAY: $57 per hour!!

Travel packages are also available for those who qualify.
If interested, email northjersey@favoritestaffing.com or call/text 973-975-4306!
We look forward to working with you!

Dionna DeGrazio
Recruiter - Northern NJ
Favorite Healthcare Staffing, Inc.

Phone/Text : (973) 975-4306
 Fax: (973) 975-4307
Email: northjersey@favoritestaffing.com

www.ingramcontent.com/pod-product-compliance
Lightning Source LLC
Chambersburg PA
CBHW021902170526
45157CB00005B/1928